The Breath of Life:
Integral Yoga® Pranayama
LEVEL I AND LEVEL II

❦

Step-by-step instructions
in the yogic breathing practices
by Sri Swami Satchidananda

Books by Sri Swami Satchidananda

Beyond Words
Enlightening Tales
The Golden Present
The Healthy Vegetarian
Heaven on Earth
Integral Yoga Hatha
Kailash Journal
To Know Your Self
The Living Gita
Meditation
The Yoga Sutras of Patanjali

Books About Sri Swami Satchidananda

Boundless Giving
Portrait of a Modern Sage
Sri Swami Satchidananda: Apostle of Peace
The Master's Touch

For a complete listing of publications, audio, and video: Shakticom.org

ISBN 978-1-938477-26-3

Printed in the United States of America on recycled text stock.

Integral Yoga® Publications, Satchidananda Ashram–Yogaville®, Inc.
108 Yogaville Way, Buckingham, Virginia, USA 23921
www.yogaville.org

The Breath of Life:
Integral Yoga® Pranayama
LEVEL I AND LEVEL II

❀

Step-by-step instructions
in the yogic breathing practices
by Sri Swami Satchidananda

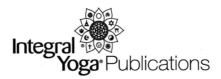

Satchidananda Ashram–Yogaville®, Inc.
Buckingham, Virginia

DEDICATION

This booklet is dedicated to our revered Master,
Sri Gurudev Swami Satchidananda Maharaj,
with abundant love and devotion.
We are immensely thankful to Sri Gurudev
for imparting the teachings of Integral Yoga
and the practices of *pranayama*
to his most grateful students.

ACKNOWLEDGMENTS

We gratefully acknowledge those
who helped this project come to fruition:

The Harry & Padma Wadhwani Family
Patrons

Swami Karunananda Ma
Project Contributor and Editor

Reverends Lakshmi and Paraman Barsel
Reverend Jivana Heyman
Project Consultants

Coleen Vimala Patterson
Graphic Design

Joelle Pearson
Copy Editor

Reverend Prem Anjali, Ph.D.
Project Designer and Manager

Contents

INTRODUCTION

The Breath of Life

*"Quite other than this physical sheath that consists
of food and interior to it is the energy sheath that
consists of breath. This is encased in the physical
sheath and has the same form. The one is filled
with the other. This first has the likeness of a
human being, and because it has the likeness of a
human, the second follows it and itself takes on
the likeness of a human. Through this vital sheath
the senses perform their office. From this humans
and beasts derive their life. For breath is the life of
beings and so is called 'the life of all.'"*
~ Taittriya Upanishad, II.2

Yoga is a world-renowned and ancient science of human
development and spiritual unfolding. The word "Yoga"
literally means "to yoke, bind, or unite." Yoga masters
have given a great deal of attention to *pranayama* as both
a healing and spiritual practice because of its benefits.
Pranayama literally translated means restraint or control
(*ayama*) of the life force (*prana*). By controlling the breath,
the Yoga practitioner is able to control the *prana*—not only
within, but also without. This leads the student toward
mastery of the body and mind, as well as higher states of
spiritual evolution.

Yoga science was systematized approximately 5,000 years ago by a sage named Patanjali and is available in a text called, the *Yoga Sutras of Patanjali*. The *Yoga Sutras* consist of 196 aphorisms that are divided into four chapters.

These aphorisms elaborate an eight-limb system of development for stilling the mind and realizing the Self. These stages are (1) *yama* or moral observances, (2) *niyama* or rules for self-purification, (3) *asana* or physical postures, (4) *pranayama* or breath regulation, (5) *pratyahara* or discipline of the senses, (6) *dharana* or concentration, (7) *dhyana* or meditation, and (8) *samadhi* or absolute tranquility.

According to the *Yoga Sutras*, a veil of mental darkness covers the light within. The benefit of *pranayama* is that it removes this veil, and the mind becomes clear and fit for concentration. While *pranayama* helps improve physical health and well-being, that is a secondary benefit; the main benefit is control of the waves of the mind through regulation of the *prana*.

CHAPTER 1

Basic Theory

Prana: The Vital Force

Prana is the vital force that makes up the entire cosmos; it is the *Parashakti*, or cosmic power. When you breathe, in addition to the oxygen, you also take in a lot of *prana*. The oxygen gets diffused in the lungs and then gets into the bloodstream, while the *prana* goes throughout the body. It enters into every area—physical, vital, and mental. Every cell of your body vibrates with new life.

You get *prana* from food, from the sun, and from the air you breathe. You can live for many weeks without food, days without water, minutes without air, but not even for a fraction of a second without *prana*.

Pranayama is the regulation of *prana*, or the life force. Breath is the external manifestation of *prana*. Thus, by regulating the breath, one can gain mastery over the *prana* within and without.

When we gain mastery over *prana*, we have mastery over the inner nature, too, because it is the *prana* that creates all the movements in an individual—physical and mental. We try to control the inner nature, because it is nature's movement that causes a lot of disturbance in the system and makes it impossible for the light within to shine in its true, original way. The body is the microcosm and the universe outside is the macrocosm. So by the regular practice of *pranayama*, we are able not only to control and direct the *prana* that functions within us, but the universal *prana* as well.

Yogic Breathing

With proper *pranayama* you begin to use the entire lungs. You can take in much more than your normal quota of oxygen and *prana*. It can be measured in laboratory tests. In a normal breath, you inhale 500 cubic centimeters of air and then breathe out the same.

After your exhalation, the lungs are almost empty, but still there is residual air in the lungs. After you breathe out your normal 500 cubic centimeters, if you pull your abdomen in slightly, you can exhale some more air, which has been measured as 1600 cubic centimeters.

After this type of full exhalation, if you begin to inhale, you first breathe in the air that you squeezed out (i.e., 1600 cubic centimeters). Then you inhale your normal 500. Then after that, you can inhale some additional air.

If you inhale more deeply, you can take in another 1600 cubic centimeters. And, after a complete squeezing out on the exhalation, you can inhale 3700 cubic centimeters. So, instead of the usual 500 cubic centimeters you would take in during a normal breath, you are taking in more than seven times as much.

If in every breath you can take in seven times more air, imagine how much more oxygen and more *prana* you will take in if you practice *pranayama* regularly.

Benefits of *Pranayama*

During *pranayama* you are literally drinking in gallons and gallons of vitality and immunity. You supercharge the blood with extra oxygen. When you retain the breath, you literally inject more oxygen into the bloodstream.

Oxygen is life, so that means you are enriching your blood with a lot of life. And not only do you take in more oxygen, but along with the air you take in more *prana*. Every cell of your body vibrates with new life. At that point no virus can even think of coming near you. As soon as it comes near, you burn it out.

That is the beauty of *pranayama*. Oxygen is a great panacea; *prana* is the best tonic—the best medicine for all kinds of poisons and viruses. Proper breathing can heal!

Pranayama also purifies the nervous system and eliminates toxins from the body and blood. It produces lightness of body, alertness of mind, good appetite, proper digestion, and sound sleep. It helps in curing asthma and other respiratory disorders. With proper breathing, you can eliminate excess mucous that causes most hay fever and sinus discomfort.

Pranayama can be used to bring heat to the body when it is cold or to cool it off when there is too much heat. You can exhilarate the blood circulation and stimulate the entire body quickly.

The quickest way to regenerate forces during the workday is through proper relaxation and deep breathing. *Pranayama* can even help improve athletic performance, because it charges the body with extra energy and builds stamina and endurance. It can help vocalists, because it expands the chest and lung capacity.

For those who wish to lose weight, *pranayama* can help reduce physical food consumption. You won't feel like overeating, because you get all the nourishment you need from the *prana* itself. For those who are trying to stop smoking, *pranayama* is the ideal practice. It helps eliminate toxins from the system, reduces the craving for nicotine, and revitalizes the lungs and body by the increased intake of oxygen.

The Yoga Energy System

The yogic science also discusses the flow of *prana* in relation to the human nervous system, and its relationship to another system of subtle nerve centers known as *nadis* and *chakras*. These *nadis* and centers are central to the process of human transformation and enlightenment. *Nadis* are channels or tubes through which blood, water, vital fluids, etc. flow in the physical body. They also have their counterpart in the other *koshas* and carry *pranic*, spiritual, and other vital energies.

Siva Samhita, the ancient scripture of Swara Yoga speaks of 350,000 *nadis*. Of these *nadis*, 14 are noted as the most important. The nervous system can be compared to a huge power-generating center. The brain and spinal cord can be seen as the generating station. The nerves and *nadis* carry the electricity throughout the body. If there is a good flow of electricity (i.e., energy or *prana*) and if the wires conducting the electricity are all strong, sturdy, and in good shape, everything runs well. But if there is not adequate flow of energy or if the wires leading from the generator are damaged or there are loose connections, then the power system does not function optimally. Through Yoga practice, particularly *pranayama*, the *nadis* and nerve centers are purified and stimulated, and the energy is channeled to optimal output and functioning.

The Five *Koshas*

Yoga texts describe five bodies or sheaths through which the human being functions. These are known as *koshas* and include the body of physical elements, the vital body, the mental body, the intellectual body, and the bliss body. Yoga practice leads the student from the grosser levels (i.e., physical body) up through the more subtle levels until bliss is reached.

When working with the breath, it is the *pranamaya kosha* (i.e., vital body) that you are handling. When you learn to regulate the *prana* and make it function the way you want, then you go to the *manomaya kosha* and regulate the mind or the thoughts.

Pranic Healing and Visualization

Adepts and highly evolved yogis have observed that the breath reflects the condition of the mind and it is a very accurate gauge of one's mental state. When agitated, for example, a person's breathing will be very shallow and quick. In the face of fear we often breathe heavily or even hold the breath. When sad or depressed, there will be a deep, sighing breath. It was discovered that by changing the breathing patterns, the mind was also affected and changed.

You can direct your *prana* with your thoughts. The breath and the mind are so intertwined that wherever one goes, the other follows. By sending your thoughts to an affected area, you send your *prana*. That is the secret behind self-healing.

When you do the deep breathing, feel that you are inhaling a lot of *prana*, a lot of vital energy. Hold your breath for a few seconds, while thinking that the *prana* is going directly to the place that aches and is building it up by removing the dead or diseased cells and tension. Then when you exhale, feel that you are throwing out all of the illness. You can feel that with the inhalation fresh energy comes in, and with the exhalation the collected toxins are thrown out. By doing this, you may be able to cure many of the aches and pains in the body, as well as long-standing illnesses. *Prana* has that power.

You can create your own imagery. Choose whatever feels comfortable. Visualization is a form of meditation, because whatever you visualize, your entire mind will focus on. You can achieve tremendous things with visualization. As you do your *pranayama* practice you can visualize light or energy. It can be energy from the sun, the stars, the moon, the ocean, or from God. The energy can be in the form of light or air or cool water. Feel that you are inhaling energy or light, and feel that flooding into your system. Feel the healing vibrations—healing energy flowing in and through your body and mind as you breathe deeply.

You can visualize light or energy in the form of streams of water or the ocean, flowing in and out, cleansing every part of the system. Feel the water come in through your head as you inhale, and then visualize the energy going directly to the needed areas. As you exhale see the toxins or any negativity all being collected and washing out. See the water washing in and washing out. See light and *prana* being infused and your entire system built up. Then as you exhale, imagine that all the unwanted things are being flushed out. As you inhale and exhale, your entire system is being charged with new energy.

Another visualization you can try is to imagine a divine being, your favorite saint, or your own Higher Self. Visualize the image of that divine being standing in front of you, blessing you. From their palms, energy is pouring toward you. As you inhale, draw in that energy and allow that divine blessing to infiltrate every cell of your system, and then while you exhale feel gratitude and thankfulness. Feel the flow of divine energy throughout your system.

Feel you are surrounded by all the great saints and sages; they are gazing at you and showering their energy and blessing upon you. Take this in through your breathing.

You can also combine your breathing with the silent repetition of a mantra or any holy name. As you inhale, you can repeat the entire mantra and exhale the same. Or you can divide the mantra between the inhalation and exhalation.

For example, you can repeat *Om* as you inhale and *Shanti* as you exhale. When you repeat the mantra, feel that it has a lot of beautiful vibrations that are resonating within you and producing tremendously healing sound vibrations in you.

Imagine that just as sound waves are used to clean jewels, the sound vibrations of the mantra are cleansing the body and mind. You can try repeating the affirmation: "These holy vibrations are flowing through me and are transforming me."

You may choose whatever visualization is most appealing to you and utilize that in your regular practice of *pranayama*. Align yourself with the Cosmic Energy, the *prana*, the Cosmic Consciousness and allow yourself to be filled and revitalized as you drink in literally gallons and gallons and gallons of vitality. *Prana* is a tonic, an elixir that builds up your physical, mental, and spiritual strength.

A capable healer can even send his or her *prana* to another person. By storing it up in the system, one can pass it on to someone in need. A person who really lives a beautiful life, who is fit and healthy, could accumulate a lot of vital energy. And by thinking or by seeing, he or she can pass that *prana* to others.

Pranayama can be a master key in unlocking the gateway to the subtle realm of self-healing, mastery of the mind, and spiritual unfolding.

Conserving *Prana*

Even as you take more *prana* in, please save and store it by regulating your life. *Prana* is wasted in many ways. The more movement in the body and mind, the more *prana* you lose. If you talk too much, without any purpose, you waste a lot of *prana*. By overeating you waste a lot of *prana*. Anything that you overdo or overindulge in results in wastage of *prana*.

The ancient yogis carefully measured how much *prana* is used by the different activities and determined that the maximum amount is expended by unlimited sex. For this reason, sexual moderation is very important. If you are moderate in sexual activities and in all areas of your life, your energy will not be depleted and your vitality will be preserved.

CHAPTER 2

Practical Guidelines

Recommended Sitting Postures for *Pranayama*

Any sitting posture may be used for performing *pranayama* as long as the spine is erect and the hands rest on the knees. However, it is optimal if one of the meditation postures (see photos) is assumed. The main meditative poses are *Padmasana* (Lotus Pose) and *Swastikasana* (Favorable Pose). The practice of *Ujjayi pranayama*, though, may be done even while standing or walking.

However you are seated—either in a chair, on a cushion, or on the floor—please make sure that the legs are comfortable and that the spine is completely erect. The head should be straight, the shoulders back, but relaxed. Arms should be gently placed on the knees, or at your side, and relaxed. Make sure there is no tension or leaning to any one side. A straight, steady posture is ideal. If the posture is crooked, a lot of the benefit will be lost and it can be harmful to do *pranayama*. While inhaling, the chest is forced to expand, and if simultaneously the crooked posture restricts it, the system undergoes strain.

To know that you are sitting straight when in a cross-legged posture, feel that your entire bodyweight is falling on your buttocks. If you are leaning back too much, there

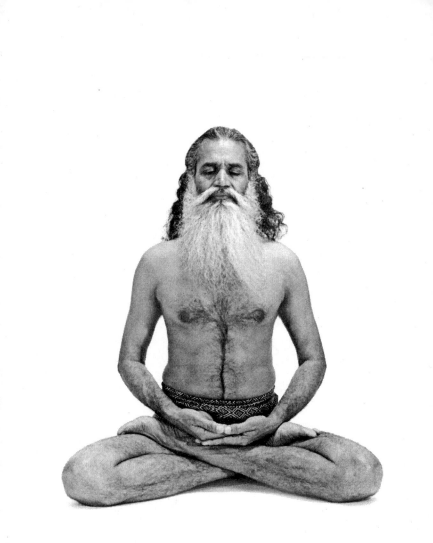

Padmasana or the Lotus Pose

will be somewhat of a gentle feeling of lifting up the knees. If you are leaning forward, you will feel a little extra weight on the knees. So, you should be seated like a triangle with the weight equally distributed.

The body should be fully relaxed. Tension means there is a wastage of *prana* and distraction of the mind to the area of tension. When the body is relaxed and the spine is erect, the subtle energy can easily flow and awaken the forces within. If at any time during your practice you feel any tension in the body, you can gently stretch out and then resume a straight and steady posture once again.

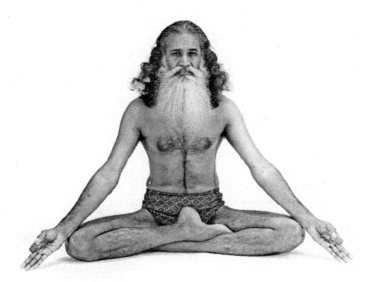

Swastikasana or the Favorable Pose

When to Practice

Prana can never be polluted by anything. So even if the air around you is polluted, that's no excuse not to practice *pranayama*. Between 4 am to 6 am, the ozone is more abundant. That's one of the reasons we recommend this as a wonderful time to practice *pranayama*, and it's also the best time to practice meditation.

Pranayama is an excellent preparation for meditation. Since the mind and the breath are closely related, you can calm the mind by regulating the breath. Do three to five rounds of rapid breathing (either *Kapalabhati* or *Bastrika*), followed by five to ten minutes of alternate nostril breathing (either *Nadi Suddhi* or *Sukha Purvaka*). Your selection will depend on whether or not you are ready for retention in your practice.

The rapid breathing energizes and awakens the system, while the alternate breathing calms and focuses the mind. The result is a very alert, yet calm and centered mind, which is ideal for meditation.

Pranayama should also be done after *asana* practice. If you are really busy, you can reduce the number of *asanas*, but *pranayama* should always be included in your practice. That is very important. *Pranayama* and meditation are food for the soul. So after the *asanas*, spend some time in deep relaxation, and then do several rounds of rapid breathing, followed by a period of alternate nostril breathing. Other breathing techniques can also be done, but rapid and alternate nostril breathing are the main ones and should always be included.

For improving one's health, it's good to have three sessions of *pranayama* daily, focusing on the rapid and alternate nostril breathing practices. Gradually develop your capacity so you can comfortably practice for 30 minutes in a session.

Pranayama should never be practiced soon after eating. Wait at least several hours until the stomach feels light. It should also never be done in strong, direct sunlight, or if you feel too tired or exhausted.

How to Practice

The earth has a gravitational force. It draws everything toward it. Your body is part of the earth. The entire body grows out of earthly elements so there is a close affinity between your body and the earth. When you do *pranayama* or meditate you can stop the magnetic pull that the earth exerts on you by insulating your body. That is why it is often recommended that you sit on a wooden plank or a folded blanket when doing these practices.

Except for the two cooling breaths, all the breathing is done through the nose, not the mouth. The nose performs many functions that aid respiration, among them: warming, moisturizing, and filtering the air. If one or both of the nostrils are blocked, you can try some *Jala Neti* (nasal cleansing) before doing *pranayama*. This can be done once daily, and the technique is described at the end of this section.

During *pranayama*, concentration should be inward to observe what is happening. On the inhalation and exhalation, concentrate on the flow of the breath and try to keep it smooth and even. During retention, just look within and see what is happening. For each person it will be different. Be conscious of the great benefits of taking in and preserving *prana* as you practice.

All retention should always be done at the throat, not at the nose, even if the nose is blocked. For the retention in

Sukha Purvaka, the pressure should not be felt at the nose, but at the throat. The greatness and benefit of *pranayama* lie in the controlled exhalation. So try to always have the exhalation slow, smooth, and controlled. If retention is done beyond one's capacity, the exhalation cannot be easy.

The ancient yogis measured how much vitality was wasted by our different activities. They determined that the faster and further the breath traveled from the body, the greater the wastage of *prana*. For this reason, they concluded that the exhalation, in particular, should not be done fast.

This is the reason why we regulate the exhalation more and do it slowly during the *pranayama* practice. The slower the exhalation, the shorter the distance the breath travels from the body, and the less *prana* is wasted.

You should always use your discretion and practice only according to your capacity. Stop and rest if ever you feel any strain. Regular practitioners who wish to have an extended *pranayama* session, including all the techniques, can use the following guidelines. However, at all times, be sure that you do not strain or go beyond your capacity.

ORDER	TIME
Nadi Suddhi	3-5 minutes
Kapalabhati	3 rounds
Bastrika	3 rounds
Sitali	5 rounds
Sitkari	5 rounds
Sukha Purvaka	10-15 minutes
Brahmari	3 minutes

As your practice develops, you can reduce the amount of time spent in *Nadi Suddhi* and *Kapalabhati* and spend more time in *Sukha Purvaka* and *Bastrika*.

Please note that *Deergha Swasam* and *Ujjayi* are not listed separately, as they can be incorporated into *Nadi Suddhi* and *Sukha Purvaka*.

Nasal Cleansing

Jala Neti or water *Neti*, helps to prevent colds and cleanses the nasal passages. It can be done with the help of a *Neti* pot, a small pot with a spout on the end designed specifically for this practice.

You can also use a teacup or the palm of your hand to hold the water you will use. Use warm (body temperature) salt water (1/2 teaspoon per cup). If you are using a *Neti* pot, as you lean over the sink, tilt your head to one side and pour the water solution in the upper nostril and let it run out of the other.

Then, reverse and pour the water into the other nostril. You can also tilt your head back, pour the water into each nostril, and spit it out through the mouth.

If using a cup or if you are cupping water in the palm of your hand, lean over a sink and tilt your head to one side, close the upper nostril with one finger and then draw in the water through the lower nostril into the mouth. Spit out the water and then repeat this process on the other side.

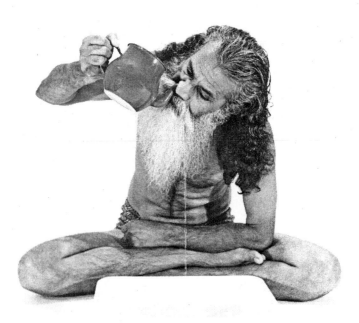

Jala Neti (Water Neti)

Warning

To derive the maximum benefit, go slowly in developing your practice. Be patient. *Pranayama* should never be done in a hurry, nor should you try to advance too quickly because you are dealing with vital energy. The Yoga scriptures personify *prana* as the deadly cobra. So remember, you are playing with a cobra. *Pranayama* is a very powerful practice that can bring certain extraordinary powers. One should adhere to certain moral and ethical principles and have good control over the mischievous mind, so as to avoid being tempted to misuse these powers. Therefore, *pranayama* should be approached carefully. Because you are dealing with such delicate organs as the lungs, the heart, and the nerve centers, you should take great care not to strain any part of the system by overdoing your practice. Do everything gently, avoid even the slightest strain, and never hurry. When practiced faithfully, with full attention toward all the instructions given, you will safely derive great benefits from your practice.

SPECIAL NOTE TO WOMEN: We recommend that women suspend the rapid breathing practices (*Kapalabhati* and *Bastrika*) during their menstrual period and also for two or three days afterward. Pregnant women who are regular practitioners may continue to practice for about the first three months, but leave out *Kapalabhati* and *Bastrika* thereafter. After childbirth, considering the condition of the body, women may restart *Kapalabhati* and *Bastrika* after the fourth or fifth month. For pregnant women who are new to Yoga but want to practice *pranayama*, we suggest only some gentle deep breathing and gentle *Nadi Suddhi* during pregnancy and for six months after childbirth.

AGE: At all ages and in all conditions of the body—stiff, tense, flabby, etc.—you can start practicing *pranayama*. However, if you have high blood pressure or coronary disease, you should not even practice *Kapalabhati* or *Bastrika* without first consulting your physician. These practices are in no way intended as a substitute for medical treatment, and we advise consulting your physician before beginning this or any Yoga program.

BEGINNERS: Beginners should not be in a hurry and thereby strain themselves. They should do the breathing techniques to their own capacity, without the least strain. Regular practice will gradually lead to perfection. The same warning applies to those who restart *pranayama* practice even after an interval of a few weeks.

LIMITS: Please carefully follow all the instructions in this program, particularly for retention of breath and length of practice. *Pranayama* is perhaps the most powerful and subtle practice in the entire system of Hatha Yoga, therefore it is essential to slowly and carefully develop your practice.

Chants

Pranayama is both a physical and spiritual discipline. Therefore, it is beneficial to begin and end your practice with some chanting or prayers. This will center the mind, and the vibrations will produce a calming effect upon the whole system, preparing you for your practice and your activities throughout the day.

A Guided Relaxation Experience

There are many things we do in life that deplete our *prana*. One of the things that debilitates the system most is stress. After finishing a set of *asanas* or before beginning *pranayama*, it is helpful to have some time for deep relaxation of the body. During this practice, stress may be easily released from the body and the system prepared to optimally benefit from the breathing practices.

To prepare for this profound relaxation experience, you will need to find a clean and quiet place where you can leave all your cares and concerns behind. Lie down on your back on a comfortable but firm mat. Have your legs about a foot apart. Let your arms be relaxed and about a foot away from your sides, with the palms facing toward the ceiling. You may now shift your body slightly until you find the position that is absolutely comfortable and most restful for you.

You will be tensing and relaxing various parts of the body. You will find that you receive maximum benefit from this, if you put all your attention into each part of the body as you tense and relax it. When you raise a part of your body, (for example your arms) please raise them slightly—perhaps six inches or less. Then when you release, just let them fall to the floor as if they were attached to a string held from above, and the string had just been cut.

First, have a few slow, deep breaths. Every time you inhale, feel that you are filling your body with total peace and tranquility. Each time you exhale, feel that you are blowing out all the tension in your body and mind. Inhale fresh cool air. Exhale hot tense air.

Now, bring your total awareness to your legs. Inhale deeply. Tense all the muscles in the legs, raise them a few inches, hold and tense a little more. And—release. Now gently roll the legs from side to side and then leave them relaxed. Just forget the legs completely.

Now we'll move on to the arms. Stretch them out, spread out the fingers of your hands. Tense. Now make each hand into a fist. Make them really tight. Inhale and raise the arms slightly and, release. Now gently roll the arms from side to side and then with the palms facing the ceiling, let them be.

Become aware of the buttocks. Inhale and tense them, holding the breath while tensing. Keep tensing—hold for a moment, and then let the tension in your buttocks and your inhalation also be suddenly released.

Now, inhale deeply through the nose, puffing up the abdomen like a balloon; take in as much air as you can, and hold the breath for a few seconds, open the mouth, and let the air gush out. Relax the abdomen. Now, inhale deeply, expanding the chest. Take in a little more air, still a little more. Hold the breath a few seconds then open the mouth and release. Relax the chest.

Become aware of your shoulders. Tighten your shoulders without moving any other part of the body. Let the shoulders be lifted and pulled toward your ears. Hold them tensed and tight. Release. Once again lift your shoulders and squeeze them tightly. Release. Now we come to the neck area. Slightly roll the head to the right and then slowly to the left. Do this a few times and as you roll the head, imagine that you are relaxing each and every muscle in your neck. Gently roll the neck, and now leave your neck relaxed and head centered. Relax the facial muscles. Tightening all the muscles in your face, squeeze them all toward the tip of the nose. Squeeze more and relax.

Now, position the body so that it is comfortable. Begin to feel a very gentle wave of relaxation coming over the entire body. Feel it coming in through the feet, coming up the legs, in through the fingers, coming up the arms. Feel the buttocks, the abdomen, and the chest relax. The relaxation continues to flow through the base of the spine, flowing through the entire back.

Now imagine this wave of relaxation, coming up to the neck, and then to the jaw and relax the chin. Feel the lips, the cheeks, and the nose relax. Feel the eyes, eyelids, and the forehead relaxing; the ears, the back of the head relaxing, and allow the last bit of tension to leave the body through the top of the head.

Allow the mind to rest and witness the peace within. This peace is your True Self; your true nature is peace. Just feel the peace and enjoy that for a few minutes. Now deepening the breath, imagine that fresh energy, *prana*, is gently entering each part of the body, starting from the head downward until the whole body is filled with vitality and is wide awake. Breathe more deeply and slowly, and please come to a comfortable seated position for the *pranayama* practice.

However you are seated, either in a chair, on a cushion or on the floor, please make sure that the legs are comfortable and that the spine is completely erect. The head should be straight, the shoulders back, but relaxed. Arms are placed to the side and relaxed or gently placed on the knees to fully expand the chest. See that there is no tension or leaning to any one side. A straight, steady posture is ideal.

If at any time you feel any tension in the body, you can gently stretch out and then resume a straight and steady posture once again.

CHAPTER 3

Pranayama Techniques: Level I

Deergha Swasam—Yogic Deep Breathing

TECHNIQUE: *Deergha Swasam* incorporates all three
levels of breathing from the diaphragm, through the
chest, and up to the clavicles or collarbones. It is complete
breathing, utilizing the full capacity of the lungs. The
three parts flow one into the next, as one complete, deep
breath. It begins with a slow exhalation through the nose.
At the end of the exhalation, pull the abdomen in slightly.

Then begin the inhalation by slowly releasing the abdomen
and allowing it to expand. Continue the inhalation as
you expand the rib cage and then continue to inhale,
allowing the upper chest to expand until the collarbones
rise slightly. The collarbones rise as the chest expands
fully, so there is no need to lift or tense the shoulders.
To exhale, reverse the order of the inhalation. First drop
the collarbones, then contract the chest, and then the
abdomen—one section flowing into the other.

For beginners, it may be easier to start part by part. To
begin the first part, exhale slowly through the nose. At the
end of the exhalation, pull the abdomen in slightly. Now
begin to inhale slowly, releasing the abdomen and allowing
it to expand. Now exhale slowly and evenly, contracting

the abdomen slightly at the end to squeeze out the last bit of air from the lungs. [Note: You can place one palm on the abdomen to help you feel its movement.]

Now add the next part. On the next inhalation, allow the abdomen to expand and then continue to inhale while expanding the chest. Now exhale fully, contracting the abdomen at the end. On the next inhalation, add the third part. So inhale, allow the abdomen, rib cage, and chest to expand and continue to inhale allowing the upper chest to expand until the collarbones rise slightly. Remember that the collarbones rise as the chest expands fully so there is no need to lift or tense the shoulders. Begin to exhale by first dropping the collarbones, then contracting the chest, and then the abdomen—one section flowing into the other. Repeat this breathing slowly and steadily.

TIME: Three to five minutes. This technique can also be practiced anytime during the day. As you progress in your practice, you can reduce the amount of time spent in *Deergha Swasam*, as the deep breathing is incorporated in the alternate nostril breathing techniques.

BENEFITS: This method of three-part deep breathing fills the lungs to capacity and empties them thoroughly, enabling you to supercharge the system with seven times as much oxygen and *prana* as in a normal breath.

Kapalabhati—The Skull Shining

TECHNIQUE: In this breathing technique, only the abdominal area will move. The chest remains still. It is particularly important during *Kapalabhati* not to slump the posture, because it is easy to strain the chest muscles if you are in the wrong position. So you may wish to place your hands on your knees, which helps to spread the chest. Be sure to keep your posture relaxed, not stiff.

Kapalabhati is rapid diaphragmatic breathing. We will do this by a series of rapid expulsions. After every expulsion the air naturally flows into the lungs and you are ready for the next expulsion. This is done in quick succession.

If you are new to this practice, it's a good idea to put your hand on the abdomen so you can feel if the abdomen moves in as the breath goes out.

When you quickly and forcefully contract the abdomen, snapping it in, automatically the air will be forcefully expelled through the nose. Then the abdomen relaxes between contractions and the air flows back in on its own.

After the last expulsion, inhale deeply and exhale as slowly as comfortable. This constitutes one round of *Kapalabhati*. Make sure your shoulders don't bounce up and down and that only the abdomen moves during *Kapalabhati*.

TIME: Beginners can begin with about three rounds of 15-20 breaths per round, and gradually over time you can build up the number of breaths per round and the number of rounds.

Experienced students can work up to five rounds of 100 or more expulsions per round, as long as there is no strain in the system.

BENEFITS: *Kapalabhati* cleanses the *nadis* in the skull and helps to burn out the excess mucous that causes sinus problems and allergies.

CAUTION: Do not hurry this breathing at any point. If dizziness results, stop the practice.

HINTS: This practice needs a firm and steady posture because of the contractions of the abdomen during the expulsions. The head, neck, and trunk should be in alignment so the chest can be well expanded and the abdominal muscles relaxed for proper breathing during this *pranayama* technique.

Nadi Suddhi—Nerve Purification

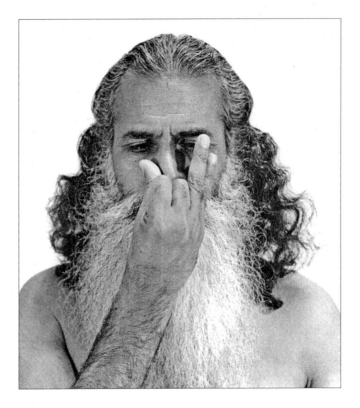

Nadi Suddhi using Vishnu Mudra

TECHNIQUE: This breath is similar to *Deergha Swasam* (the Yogic Deep Breathing) with the addition of alternating the nostrils, isolating one nostril at a time.

STAGE 1: Form *Vishnu Mudra* (see photo) in order to help alternate the nostrils. To do this, make a loose fist with the right hand. Extend the thumb and the last two fingers. [Note: If *Vishnu Mudra* is very uncomfortable, you can use the index finger and thumb of the right hand.] Close off the right nostril by pressing against the side of the nostril with the thumb. Exhale slowly and deeply through the left nostril, and then begin a deep inhalation through the same nostril.

Now close off the left nostril by pressing against the side of the nostril with the last two fingers. Release the thumb so you may exhale slowly and deeply through the right nostril. Now inhale through the right nostril. Once again, close off your right nostril with the extended thumb and begin to exhale through your left nostril.

Continue your breathing by inhaling through the same nostril and then change to the other side. The pattern is: Exhale, inhale, and switch. Exhale, inhale, and switch. Remember to make your breathing full and deep, incorporating *Deergha Swasam*, starting each inhalation by relaxing the abdomen and allowing it to expand, and continuing while expanding the rib cage, and then the upper chest until the collarbones rise slightly. Then exhaling slowly, first dropping the collarbones, then contracting the chest, and then the abdomen—one section flowing into the other. End your practice with an exhalation through the right nostril.

STAGE 2: When you feel comfortable with this practice, you can begin to make the exhalation longer than the inhalation, slowly creating a ratio of 1:2, so that the exhalation takes twice as long as the inhalation. You can begin to count the inhalations and exhalations by mentally counting, "*Om* 1, *Om* 2, *Om* 3," etc. instead of simply "1, 2, 3." This will give you an accurate count of the seconds, as well as the added beneficial vibration of repeating *Om*.

Gradually you will be able to make the exhalations twice as long as the inhalations. For example, if you inhale for three seconds—counting "*Om* 1, *Om* 2, *Om* 3"—you will exhale for six seconds—*Om* 1 to *Om* 6. If you begin your 1 to 2 ratio with a week of 3-second inhalations to 6-second exhalations, the next week you can try a ratio of 4 to 8. Practice each count until you reach 10:20—that means 10-second inhalations to 20-second exhalations. Be sure never to increase the count until you are completely comfortable with the count you are currently doing.

TIME: About three minutes to start with.

BENEFITS: *Nadi Suddhi* brings lightness of body, alertness of mind, good appetite, proper digestion, and sound sleep. The *nadis* are the subtle nerves or channels through which the *prana* flows throughout the system. By ensuring the *nadis* are clean and strong, this practice brings health and vitality to every part of the body at the most fundamental level. This practice is also extremely calming to the mind and prepares it for meditation.

CAUTION: After reaching a 10:20 count, don't increase the count, but simply increase the number of rounds per sitting. Only after you build up to 10:20 and can comfortably do 30 to 50 breaths using this ratio will you be ready for the more advanced practice of *Sukha Purvaka*.

NOTE: Keep the awareness on the flow of the breath. The more focused the mind, the more powerful and healing the practice. In order to make the breath completely silent, let there be a gentle control from the diaphragm and not the nose on both the inhalation and exhalation. See that your arm remains relaxed and not stiff, with the elbow close to the body.

Brahmari—Humming Bee

TECHNIQUE: Inhale through the nostrils, filling the lungs completely. Exhale, making a humming sound. Try and feel the vibration on the soft palate at the roof of the mouth. Feel or imagine that the vibration is going straight up through the head to the crown of the head and out into the cosmos.

TIME: Do five rounds at various pitches.

BENEFITS: *Brahmari pranayama* tones the vocal chords, creates sound vibrations for concentration, and enables us to get in touch with the *Pranava*—the primordial hum of the universe.

Pranayama Techniques: Level II

Ujjayi—Hissing Breath

TECHNIQUE: After a complete exhalation, inhale slowly and evenly while tightening the glottis. This partially closes the opening to the windpipe, so that a continuous, soft hissing sound is heard. The exhalation is done the same way, producing the hissing sound. The sound should be a soft hiss and of even pitch and intensity throughout. The sound is completely from the back of the throat and not the nose.

[Note: The sound should be quiet enough that others in the room won't be able to hear you; in this way you also preserve more *prana* in the system.]

Continue this practice, remembering to use the yogic deep breathing. By keeping the sound smooth and even, *Ujjayi* enables you to make your breath smooth, even, and slow. You can focus your mind on listening to that soft hissing sound, which helps to draw the mind inward.

TIME: There is no time restriction. The breathing should be done evenly throughout the practice. Even the least strain is to be avoided.

BENEFITS: *Ujjayi* increases the control over the breath and is an aid to concentration. It relieves heat in the head and increases the digestive fire. It can be helpful in the healing of asthma and other respiratory diseases. It adds luster to the face.

CAUTION: If this is a new practice for you, be careful not to strain or hurt the throat. You may experience some fatigue, so try it only for a few minutes each day at first. Gradually build up over time to where you can use this technique with the same slow inhalations and exhalations in all the *pranayama* practices.

Bastrika—Bellows Breath

TECHNIQUE: This is rapid breathing similar to *Kapalabhati*, but with the addition of retention of the breath. To aid in the retention of breath, we utilize *Jalandhra Bandha*, the chin lock. To perform the chin lock, take a full, deep inhalation and hold the breath while bending the neck forward, keeping the back and shoulders erect, and bring the chin as close to the chest as possible. Then lift the chin, and slowly exhale. If after the slow exhalation, the breath comes rushing in, you have held the retention too long. Remember also that retention is done at the throat, without building pressure in the nose.

During *Bastrika pranayama*, the emphasis is on the forceful exhalation caused by snapping the abdomen inward, similar to *Kapalabhati*. You also can have a slight effort on the inhalation. So there will be a series of forced exhalations, followed by slight effort on the inhalations. Each round will consist of a series of rapid expulsions and slightly forceful inhalations followed by a deep exhalation, a complete inhalation, retention with chin lock, and finally a slow, deep exhalation.

Now that you have been practicing *Kapalabhati* for a while, the rounds can be longer, and as you continue your practice, you can lengthen the rounds by adding more expulsions to each round. Retention can also be gradually lengthened, but never to the point where there is the least strain. You should always be able to do a slow deep exhalation at the end of each round, without the breath rushing out on the exhalation.

Begin now with a series of rapid expulsions and slightly forceful inhalations. End with a complete exhalation, followed by a full, deep inhalation, all the way up so the collarbones rise. Then retain the breath by bending the head and neck forward, bringing the chin as close to the chest as possible to form *Jalandhra Bandha*. Then raise the head slowly and exhale slowly and evenly through the nose using *Ujjayi*. Let the breath return to normal and relax. You can adjust the breath retention to your own capacity.

During the inhalation, exhalation, and retention with chin lock at the end of each round, you may also apply a very powerful technique that follows the breath along the spine. This will help you become conscious of the psychic energy traveling along the spine that passes through certain spiritual centers, called *chakras*.

After the last rapid expulsion, when you take a deep inhalation, try to feel that energy is coming from the crown of the head, down the spine, and striking gently at the base of the spine. While you retain the breath, see if you can feel a very mild heat or gentle warmth along the spine, which will feel very pleasant. If at first you don't feel it, just imagine that, and then gradually you will feel it. You should draw that energy up to either the heart or eyebrow center and focus on either center throughout the retention. Then, on the final exhalation, feel that the energy is flowing down to the base of the spine and then back up to the crown of the head.

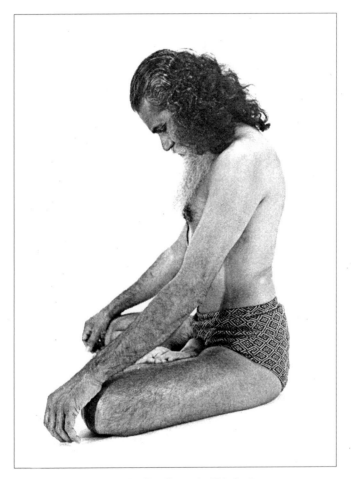

Jalandhra Bandha or the Chin Lock

TIME: Do three to five rounds of *Bastrika* with *Jalandhra Bandha*.

BENEFITS: *Bastrika* exhilarates the blood circulation and stimulates the entire body quickly. It brings heat to the body when it is cold and can be used to help keep the body warm during the winter. It improves digestion, removes phlegm, and helps in curing asthma and other respiratory problems. It builds up and strengthens the entire respiratory system, and raises energy.

CAUTION: Do not hurry this breathing at any point, nor retain the breath beyond your capacity. If the breath comes rushing out on the exhalation, then you've held the retention too long. If dizziness occurs, discontinue, and let the breath return to normal. Between rounds, take a few normal breaths.

Sukha Purvaka—Easy, Comfortable Breath

TECHNIQUE: This breath is a more advanced form of *Nadi Suddhi*, the alternate nostril breathing, because it employs retention. When you can comfortably practice *Nadi Suddhi* at a 10:20 ratio for 30-50 breaths (or 10 rounds) in a sitting, you can begin *Sukha Purvaka*. The pattern for *Sukha Purvaka* is: exhale, inhale, retain, and change nostrils; exhale, inhale, retain, and change nostrils.

Form *Vishnu Mudra* with your right hand. Close off the right nostril and exhale slowly through the left nostril for a count of 20. Then inhale for a count of 10 through the same nostril. Now close off both nostrils and retain the breath for 5 seconds. Release the thumb from the right nostril and exhale slowly and completely through the same nostril for a count of 20. Then inhale through the right nostril for a count of 10. Close off both nostrils and retain the breath for 5 seconds. Release the left nostril and exhale to a count of 20. Inhale through the left nostril for 10 seconds. Close off both nostrils and retain the breath for 5 seconds. Release the right nostril and exhale for 20 seconds. Inhale through the right nostril to a count of 10, close off both nostrils and retain for 5 seconds. Release the left nostril and exhale to a count of 20.

Continue breathing with this pattern of exhale, inhale through the same nostril and retain, then change to the other side. You may also continue this practice employing a technique that follows the breath along the spine. During the inhalation, try to feel that the energy is coming from the crown of the head, down the spine, and striking gently at the base of the spine. While you retain the breath, see if you feel a very mild heat or gentle warmth along the spine, which will feet very pleasant.

You should draw the energy up to either the heart or eyebrow center and focus on either center throughout the retention. On the exhalation, feel that the energy is flowing down to the base of the spine and then back up to the crown of the head. If you feel comfortable, you can continue *Sukha Purvaka* with this technique. Remember to end your practice with an exhalation through the right nostril.

TIME: 10-15 minutes.

BENEFITS: *Sukha Purvaka* has all the benefits of *Nadi Suddhi*, plus it enriches the quality of the blood and ensures optimal physical health. It helps the mind become clear and steady, enabling good concentration. It is an excellent preparation for meditation.

CAUTION: As you develop your practice, at no time should there be even the least strain in the system. The flow of the breath should remain slow and steady, and there should be no dizziness or discomfort.

Sitali—Cooling Breath

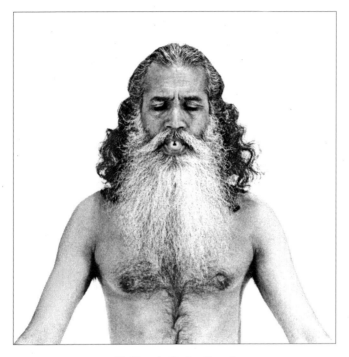

Sitali or the Cooling Breath

TECHNIQUE: To do this breathing practice, you will curl the sides of the tongue up lengthwise into a long tube. You can check the picture in the booklet to see how this should look. Also, please note that if you find it difficult to curl the tongue, you can skip over this breath, as there is a second cooling breath that everyone can easily do.

First, exhale completely through the nose. Then project the tongue out (as if sticking your tongue out), curling it up. Forcefully draw air in through the tube with a hissing sound. Fill the lungs completely. Draw the tongue inside the mouth, close the mouth, and retain the air for a few seconds. Then, exhale slowly and completely through the nose.

As you practice *Sitali*, you can concentrate on the coolness of the air on the tongue and throat, and as you retain the air, you can feel the coolness spreading through the body. After the last round, relax and allow the breath to return to normal. Feel how cooling this breath is to the entire system.

TIME: Three to five rounds.

BENEFITS: *Sitali* helps remove heat, thirst, hunger, and sleepiness. It is especially useful for dissipating the excess heat that can build up when doing the more advanced *pranayama* practices. It's also useful in hot weather.

Sitkari—Wheezing Breath

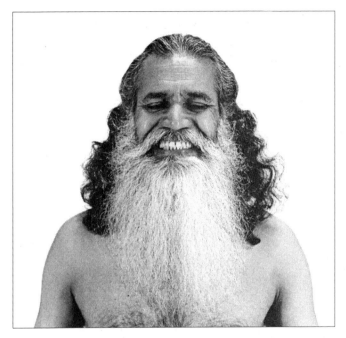

Sitkari or the Wheezing Breath

TECHNIQUE: In this practice, air is sucked in through clenched teeth, rather than through the curled tongue. Curl the tip of the tongue back so it touches the upper palate. Then open your lips and gently clench your teeth—as if you are smiling through clenched teeth. Now suck in the breath, with a deep inhalation through your clenched teeth, making a hissing sound.

Feel the air entering through either side of the mouth, and now hold the air for a few seconds. Then slowly and completely exhale through the nose. You can concentrate on the cool feeling on the gums and tongue as you do this practice. After the last round, relax and allow the breath to return to normal. Feel how *Sitkari* cools the entire system.

TIME: Three to five rounds.

BENEFITS: Similar to *Sitali* in its benefits, *Sitkari* also helps improve the health of the gums.

Brahmari with *Mudra*

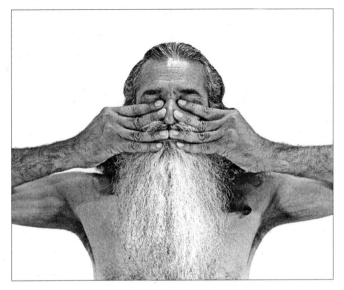

Shanmukhi Mudra or the Six-way Seal

TECHNIQUE: At the end of *Brahmari pranayama*, apply *Shanmukhi Mudra* (the Six-way Seal). This will help to introvert the mind, so you may hear the inner vibration better, which will lead you nicely into meditation. The external senses are shut out by placing both hands in *Shanmukhi Mudra* (see photo above).

After the last round of *Brahmari*, you can raise the elbows sideways to shoulder level and apply *Shanmukhi Mudra* by placing the index fingers over the lower edges of each

55

eyelid, not pressing on the eyeball at all, but just holding the eyelid shut. Then, the middle fingers will rest across the bridge of the nose. The lips are shut by placing the ring fingers above the lips and the pinky fingers beneath the lower lip and gently pressing the two together. Lastly, the thumbs close the ears, by pressing on the flap over the outside of the ear canal.

Brahmari is done by taking a deep inhalation, and on the exhalation, making a loud and resonating humming sound. Try and feel the vibration on the soft palate at the roof of the mouth. Feel or imagine that the vibration is going straight up through the head to the crown of the head and out into the cosmos. After the last round, apply the *mudra* for as long as you are comfortable and have a few minutes of silent meditation. During the meditation, you can allow the mind to focus on the lingering hum or you can just enjoy the peaceful feeling. You can also try applying the *mudra* while you are humming.

TIME: Do eight rounds at various pitches.

BENEFITS: *Brahmari* tones the vocal chords and creates sound vibrations for concentration. *Shanmukhi Mudra* is a great aid toward the practice of concentration as it helps to draw the mind inward.

APPENDIX

Closing Chant

Lokah Samastah Sukhino Bhavanthu

May the entire universe
be filled with peace and joy, love and light.

Words of Blessing from
Sri Swami Satchidanandaji Maharaj

There is no better health tonic than
Yoga *asanas* and *pranayama*.
Remember: Health is your birthright, not disease;
strength is your heritage, not weakness;
courage, not fear; bliss, not sorrow;
peace, not restlessness;
knowledge, not ignorance.

May you attain this birthright, this divine heritage,
to shine as fully developed yogis.
May the great science of *pranayama*
bring you radiant health, a balanced mind,
and a dedicated life filled with all divine energy,
so you may serve the entire creation
with peace and joy, love and light.

Om Shanti, Shanti, Shanti.

Recommended Reading

Satchidananda, Swami (2012).
The Yoga Sutras of Patanjali: Translation and Commentary.
Buckingham, VA: Integral Yoga® Publications.

Satchidananda, Swami (2011).
Meditation.
Buckingham, VA: Integral Yoga® Publications.

Satchidananda, Swami (2007).
Integral Yoga Hatha.
Buckingham, VA: Integral Yoga® Publications.

Further Resources

The Breath of Life: Integral Yoga® Pranayama is also available as an audiobook from www.shakticom.org and Integral Yoga® Distribution (www.iydbooks.com). In this 2-CD set, Sri Swami Satchidananda leads the same step-by-step instructions provided in this book.

We highly recommend that you combine your practice of *pranayama* with other Yoga practices. Integral Yoga® Hatha classes, on CD and DVD, offer instruction in the practice of *asanas*, deep relaxation, *pranayama*, and meditation. "Guided Relaxation" and "Guided Meditation" CDs offer further in-depth instruction in deep relaxation and meditation respectively, as taught by Sri Swami Satchidananda and Integral Yoga® International.

For further information on Integral Yoga® classes, publications, teachers training programs, and retreats, please call your local Integral Yoga® Institute or visit the website of the Integral Yoga® Teachers Association (www.iyta.org) for a listing of centers and Integral Yoga teachers in your area.

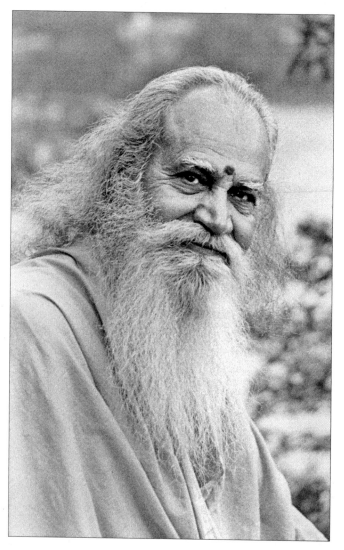

About Sri Swami Satchidananda

Sri Swami Satchidananda was one of the great Yoga masters to bring the classical Yoga tradition to the West in the 1960s. He taught Yoga postures and meditation, and he introduced students to a vegetarian diet and a more compassionate lifestyle.

During this period of cultural awakening, iconic Pop artist Peter Max and a small circle of his artist friends invited Sri Swamiji to extend an intended two-day visit to New York City so that they could learn from him the secret of attaining physical health, mental peace, and spiritual enlightenment.

Three years later, he led some half a million American youth in chanting "*Om*," when he delivered the official opening remarks at the 1969 Woodstock Music and Art Festival and became known as "the Woodstock Guru."

The distinctive teachings he brought with him integrate the physical discipline of Yoga, the spiritual philosophy of India, and the interfaith ideals he pioneered. Those techniques and concepts influenced a generation and spawned a Yoga culture that is flourishing today. Currently, more than twenty million Americans practice Yoga as a means for managing stress, promoting health, slowing down the aging process, and creating a more meaningful life.

The teachings of Sri Swami Satchidananda have entered the mainstream, and there are now thousands of Integral Yoga® teachers around the globe. Integral Yoga Institutes, teaching centers, and certified teachers throughout the United States and abroad offer classes, workshops, retreats, and teacher training programs featuring all aspects of Integral Yoga. Integral Yoga is also the foundation for Dr. Dean Ornish's landmark work in reversing heart disease and Dr. Michael Lerner's noted Commonweal Cancer Help program.

In 1979, Sri Swamiji was inspired to establish Satchidananda Ashram–Yogaville®. Founded on his teachings, it is a place where people of different faiths and backgrounds can come to realize their essential oneness. One of the focal points of Yogaville is the Light Of Truth Universal Shrine (LOTUS). This unique interfaith shrine honors the Spirit that unites all the world faiths, while it celebrates their diversity. People from all over the world come there to meditate and pray.

Over the years, Sri Swamiji received many honors for his public service, including the Juliet Hollister Interfaith Award presented at the United Nations and, in 2002, the U Thant Peace Award. On the occasion of his birth centennial in 2014, he was posthumously honored with the James Parks Morton Interfaith Award by the Interfaith Center of New York. In addition, he served on the advisory boards of many Yoga, world peace, and interfaith organizations. He is the author of numerous books on Yoga and he is the subject of the documentary, *Living Yoga: The Life and Teachings of Swami Satchidananda*.

For more information: www.swamisatchidananda.org and www.integralyoga.org

NOTES

NOTES